David, Donny, and Darren

Virginia Totorica Aldape
Photographs by Lillian S. Kossacoff

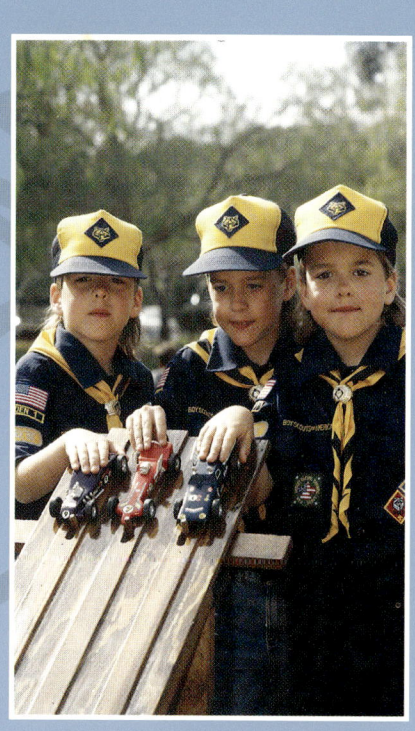

LERNER PUBLICATIONS COMPANY / MINNEAPOLIS

To David and Diana Berggren, and to all the parents of multiples.
                                    —Virginia Aldape

To motherhood and family. To Brett and SMB.
                                    —Lillian Kossacoff

Illustrations by John Erste

Text copyright © 1997 by Virginia Totorica Aldape
Photographs copyright © 1997 by Lillian S. Kossacoff

LIBRARY OF CONGRESS CATALOGING-IN-PUBLICATION DATA

Aldape, Virginia Totorica.
     David, Donny, and Darren : a book about identical triplets /
Virginia Totorica Aldape ; photographs by Lillian S. Kossacoff.
        p. cm.
     Includes bibliographical references.
     ISBN 0-8225-2584-4 (alk. paper)
     1. Triplets—Juvenile literature. 2. Multiple birth—Juvenile literature.
I. Kossacoff, Lillian S. II. Title.
GN63.6.A43   1997
306.875—dc20   96-33551

Manufactured in the United States of America
1 2 3 4 5 6 – JR – 02 01 00 99 98 97

CONTENTS

As you read the story, try to identify who's who in each photo.
If you need help, turn to this page for the answers.

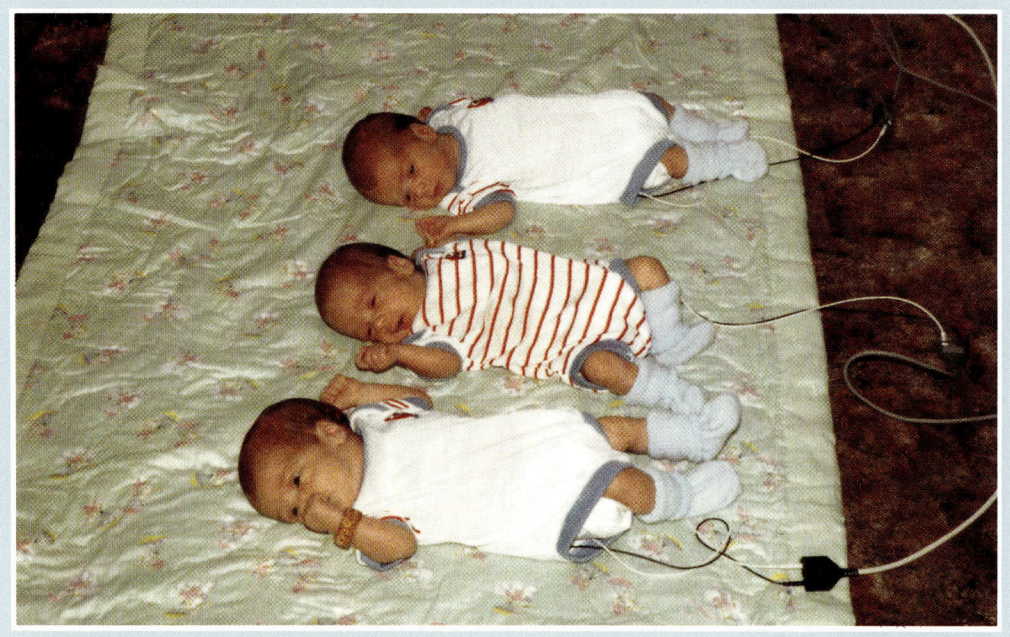

ON THE DAY WE WERE BORN, we surprised everyone. We arrived two months early. And to top it off, Mom thought she was having twins.

Mom and Dad have told us the story many times. After two of us were born, the doctor said to our mom, "You have two fine, beautiful boys." Then he put my brothers, David and Donny, in incubators.

Suddenly, a second doctor said, "Here's a surprise!"

"Oh my!" said the primary doctor. "We have a *C*."

"What's a *C*?" Mom asked.

"A *C* is baby number three," said the doctor. "You have triplets!"

"Show me," Mom said. The doctors held up all three of us.

After we were born, the nurse came to the waiting room to talk with our family. Everyone was worried about Mom because she had been so sick on the way to the hospital.

"Mr. Mason," said the tired nurse.

"What's wrong?" Dad asked.

"You have triplets," she said with a smile.

Grandpa's heart fluttered. Dad almost fainted. Grandma really fainted. No one could believe that Mom had given birth to triplets. David and Donny each weighed 3 pounds 13 ounces. I weighed 3 pounds 6 ounces. We were all 11 inches long. That's as long as the paper in your notebook.

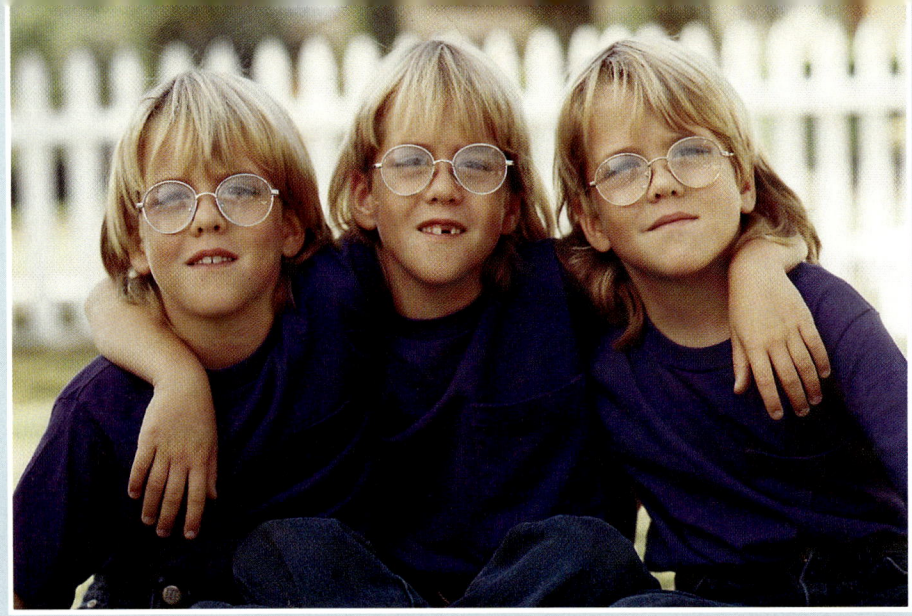

Now we are eight years old, and we can talk about
what it's like to be identical triplets. We look very much
alike. Our hair is blond. We have brown eyes. We wear
glasses with the same prescription, so we can trade them if
we want. We even smile alike, sometimes.

When people can't tell us apart, my brothers and I have to
tell them who we are. If someone calls me Donny or David,
I usually say, "That's not me. I'm Darren!"

Dad says the best way to tell who's who is by looking at
our faces. Donny has the fullest face. Mine is more slender.
David's face is in the middle.

When people don't know who we are by looking at our faces, they look at the colors and clothes we're wearing. David likes baggy purple pants with plaid shirts. Donny won't touch a plaid shirt. He likes to wear hats and the color blue. Donny loves jean shorts, jean pants, jean anything. I like wearing shorts, any kind of shorts. I wish I never had to wear long pants. And I like the color red.

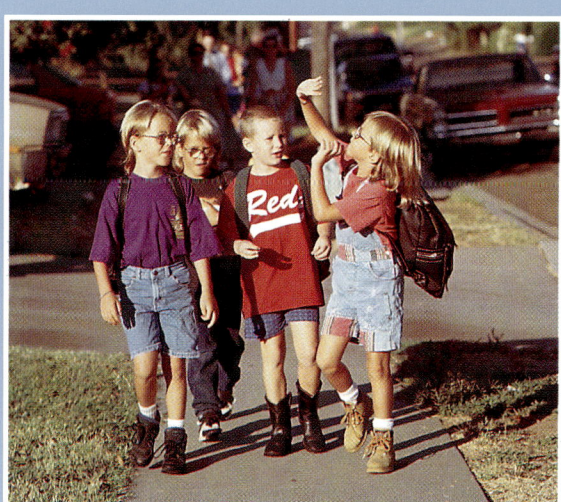

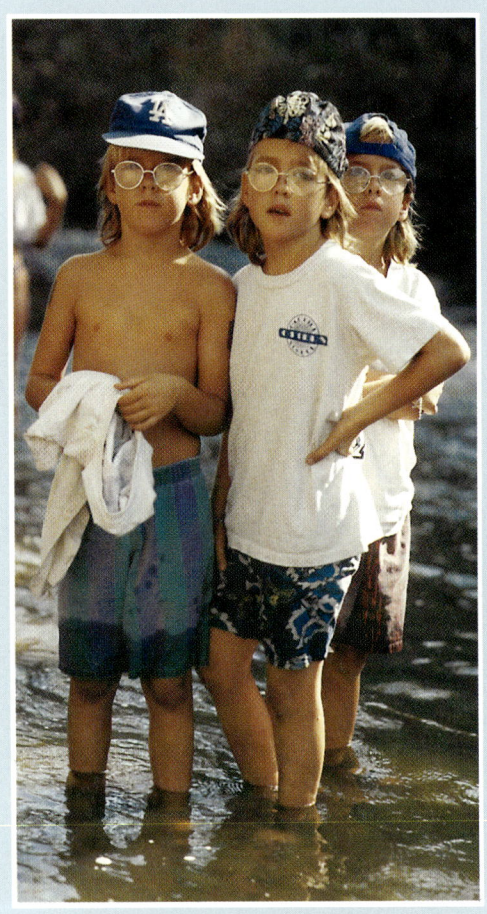

Sometimes we think people are way too curious. When we were five, a story was written about us in the local newspaper. At first we liked the story. But after a while, we didn't like it as much because people would stop and ask us questions. Once, while we were sitting in our eye doctor's office, a stranger recognized us from the article. The stranger asked, "Are you all boys?" What a dumb question. Of course we're all boys!

OFTEN KIDS AND TEACHERS can't tell us apart. One day I was sitting with Donny during lunch. One of his friends looked at us and asked, "Are *you* Donny or are *you* Donny?" I wanted to trick the friend so I said, "I'm Donny." But the friend knew our voices. He could tell it was me because Donny's voice sounds a lot tougher.

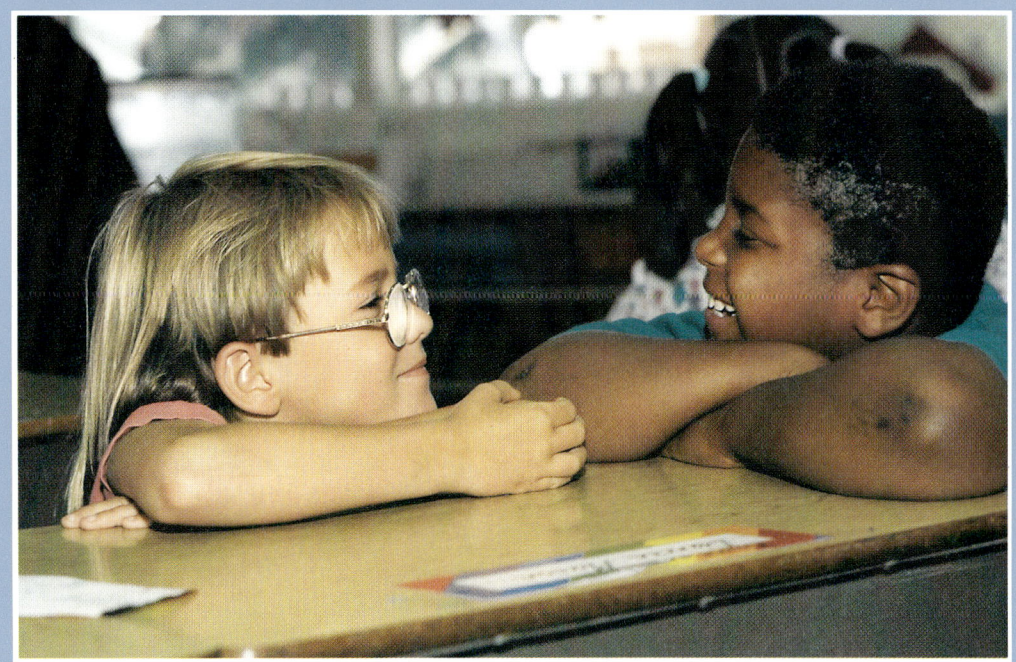

Occasionally, Mom mixes us up when she isn't paying attention. When David wore a blue shirt one day, Mom called him "Donny" all day long. We can't give Mom too hard a time, though. Once it happened to us.

One night, our family was eating dinner. I got up for some water, then Donny got up. I turned to Donny and said, "David, you need to wait until I'm done." Donny just laughed. Then I looked again and said, "Oh, no. You're Donny, not David!" We all laughed a lot.

When someone in our family mixes us up, it's okay. But we don't like it when other people don't even *try* to tell us apart. They just call out our names—David, Donny, Darren.

Mom says that whatever happens to one of us will happen to the other two within a few days. Last week, David lost one of his teeth. Two days later Donny found a hard lump in his chili. Donny asked Mom what the hard stuff was. When Mom said she didn't put anything hard in the chili, Donny looked again. "Oh, my gosh, it's my tooth!" he said. It was the tooth just like the one David lost a couple days before.

As babies, we couldn't
fall asleep unless we were
touching. Mom would place
our cribs close together so we
could put our arm or leg
through the crib bars to reach
each other. It didn't matter if it
was our big toe or one finger.
We just needed to be touching
each other. When we have
sleepovers with our friends, we
still put our sleeping bags right
together.

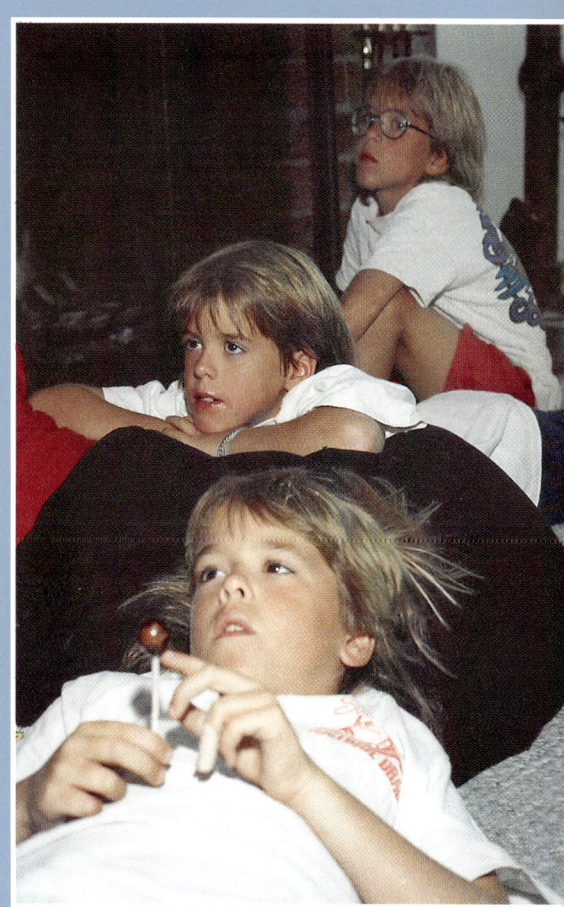

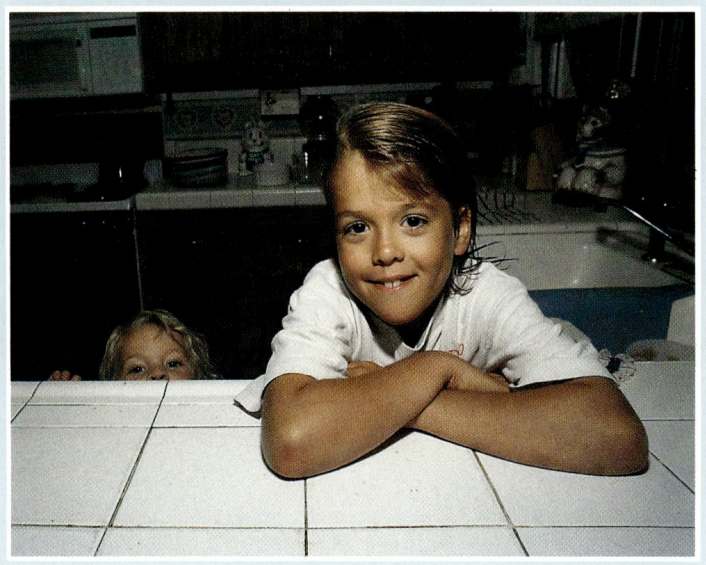

WE LIVE IN ESCONDIDO, CALIFORNIA, with our dad, our mom, and our baby brother, Pauly. Pauly is two years old and is an okay little brother. He always picks one of us to do favorite things with him. On days when Pauly wants me to be his buddy, he copies what I do. During dinner Pauly likes to sit next to Donny. They often share their food. At bedtime Donny sings Pauly a little song. Pauly picks David when he wants to snuggle in bed.

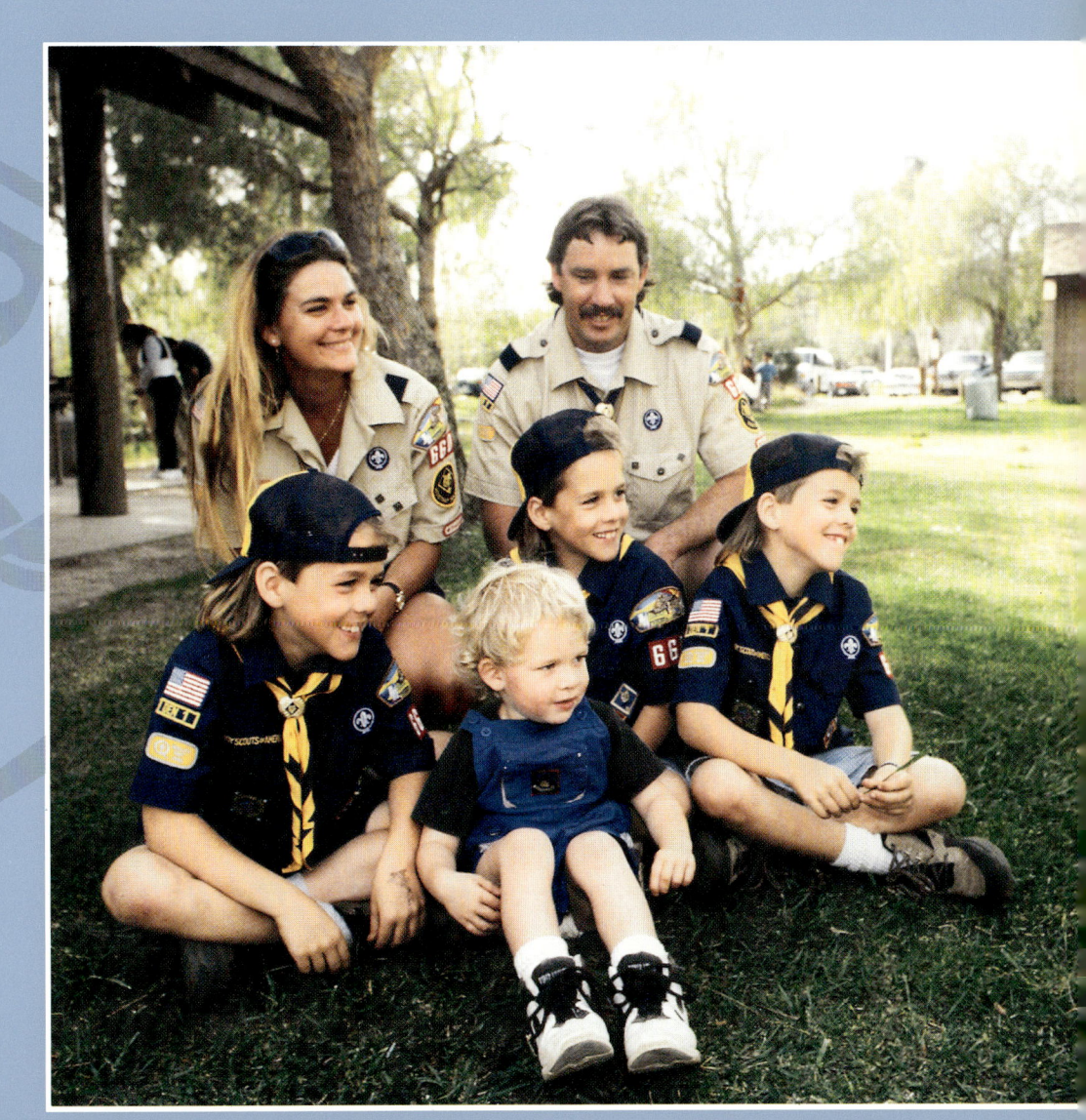

We have two dogs, Edgar and Inga. They are Rottweilers and are very protective of us. If someone comes into our yard, watch out! Edgar and Inga can tell us apart. If Mom tells Edgar to get David, Edgar will grab David's shirt and nudge him until he finds out what Mom wants. Edgar and Inga know the difference between our bedrooms, too.

We used to have a cat named Liberty. He was Mom's cat when she was a little girl. Liberty was still alive when Pauly was born. Last year when Liberty died, we buried him in the front yard.

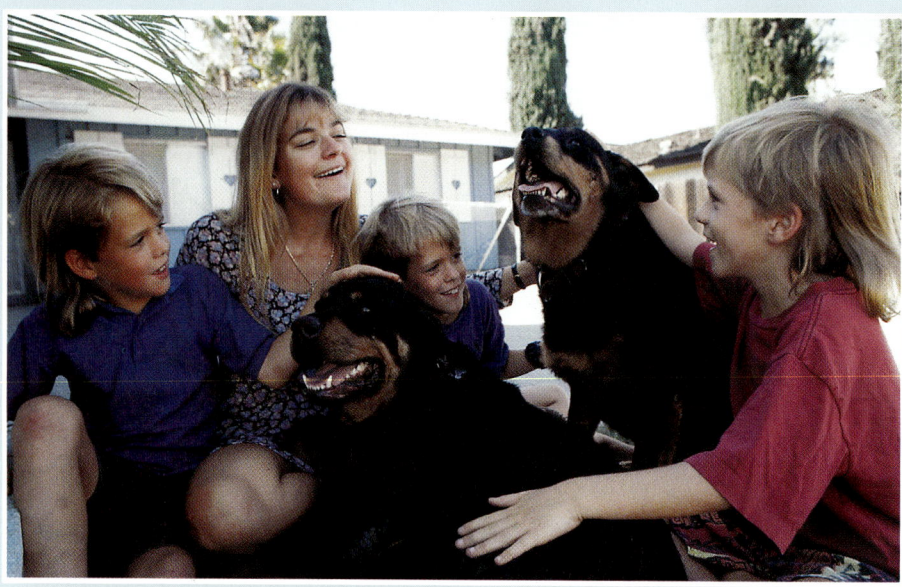

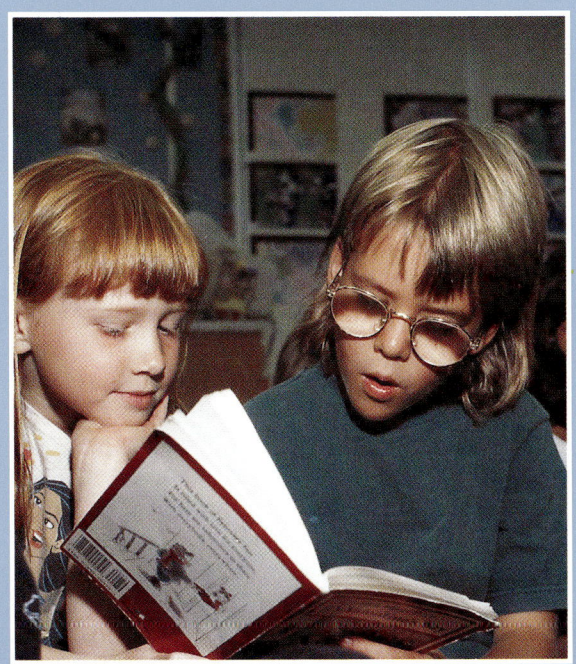

ON SCHOOL MORNINGS, Dad wakes us up at six-thirty. We take our baths at night so there's not a rush for the bathroom in the morning. We get dressed, make our beds, and pick up our rooms. We usually eat cereal for breakfast, but sometimes Mom fixes omelets or French toast. By the time Dad leaves for work, we are brushing our teeth and combing our hair. Mom walks us to school. We leave at quarter of eight, whether we're ready or not. That's our schedule.

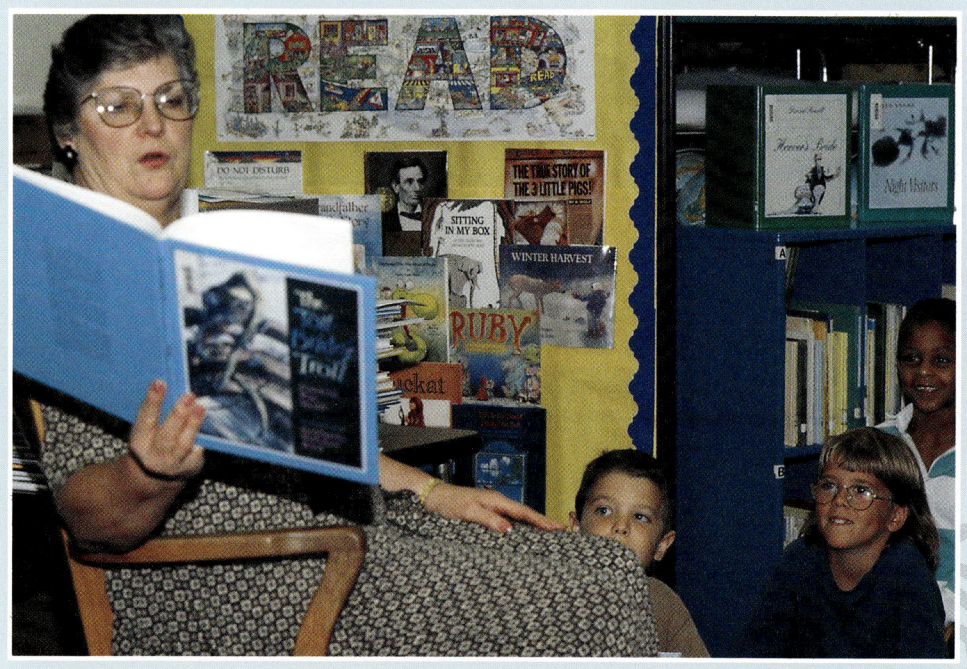

We're in second grade at Oak Hill Elementary School. We each have a different teacher. Since we were born early, the doctors told Mom not to expect us to keep up with kids our age. The doctors also said that we would probably be in special classes at school. We have surprised everyone—we like school and aren't in any special classes.

When we come home from school, we have a snack. After that, we have to do our homework. Then we do our chores. We get an allowance for doing these chores. Mom has a schedule and she helps us keep track of the jobs we need to do. We set the table, empty the dishwasher, and pick up the dog doo-doo in the yard. After our homework and chores are finished, we can finally play.

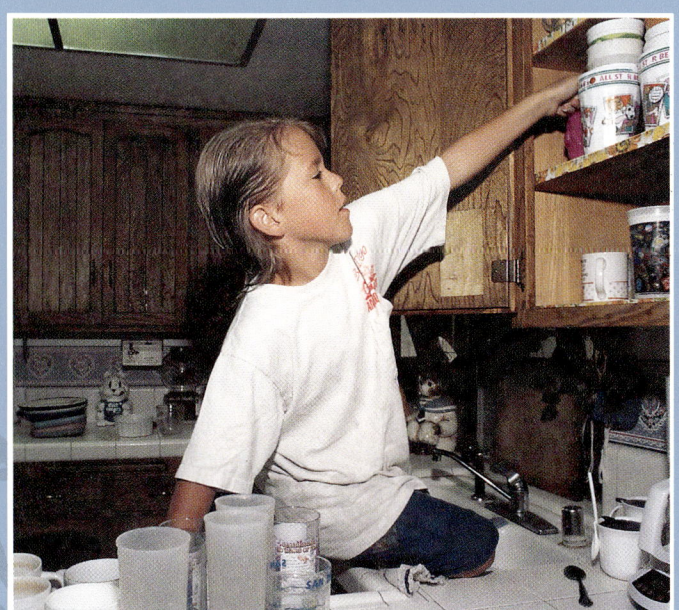

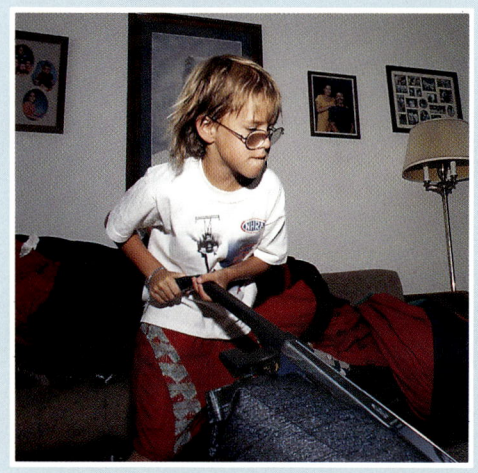
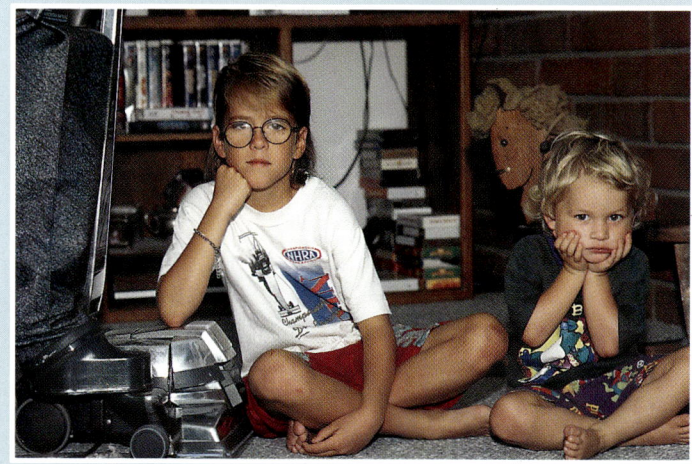

Mom gives us extra money if we sweep off the driveway, clean the bathroom, vacuum the carpet, or wash the dog bowls. If we do any of these chores without being asked, we earn an extra quarter for each job. Mom and Dad won't give us a quarter if they have to ask us to clean our dirty bedrooms—only if we do it without being told. David likes money in his pocket, so he's always looking for extra jobs.

Mom started teaching us to do our laundry when we were two years old. She taught us how to fold our clothes. Our clothes probably didn't look good, but we did it anyway.

Now we each do our own laundry. We separate the lights and the darks, start the washer, and put in the soap. When the washer's done, we put the clothes in the dryer. When the clothes are dry, we fold them and put them away. We do it all. Mom doesn't have to help us anymore.

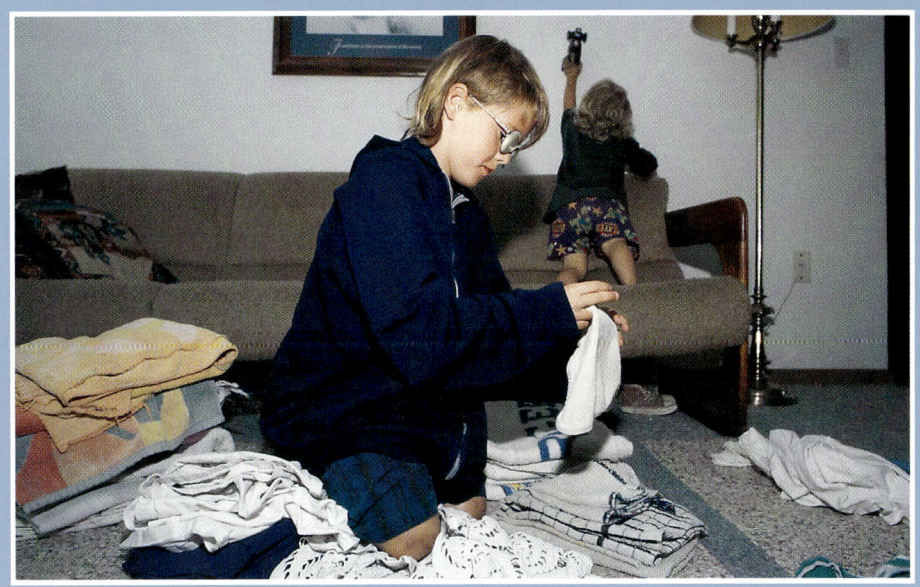

DAVID, DONNY, AND I ARE CLOSE. We like to do most things together and help each other out. A few weeks ago, we were at a friend's house. There was a tree we wanted to climb, but the lowest branch was too high for us to reach. We looked at each other and Donny said, "I'll get down on my hands and knees. You guys can climb on my back, reach the branch, and pull yourselves up. Then you can pull me up." We had fun that day.

Even though we're close, it's okay if a friend invites only one of us to go someplace. But most of our friends are friends with all three of us. That's how we like it.

We like to ride bikes, play basketball, and race derby cars together. We like to make deals with each other, too. If David gets out the cereal and the milk, sometimes he'll ask Donny or me to put them away. Or Donny will say, "David, if you do my dishes today, I'll do yours tomorrow."

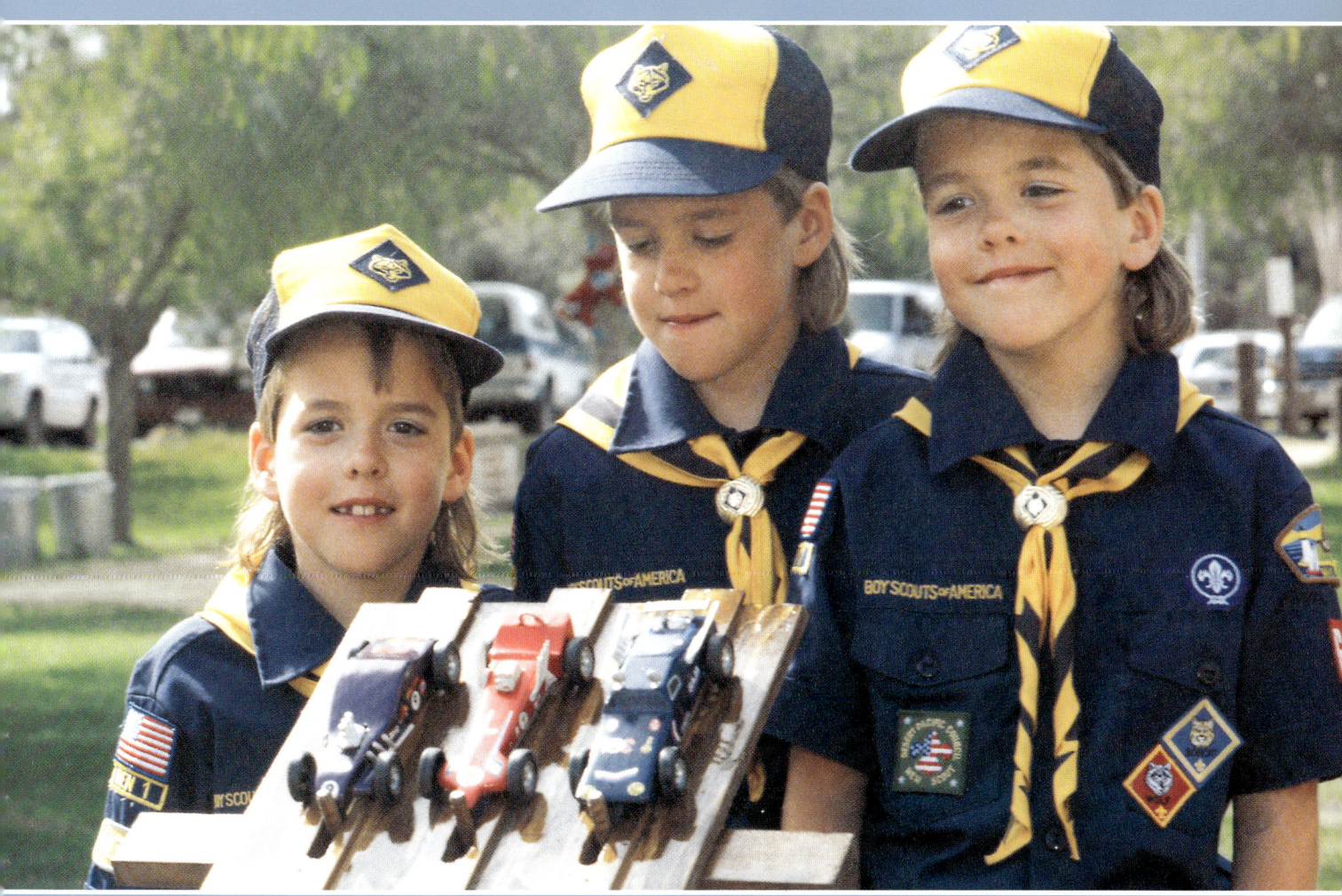

We love cooking dinner with Mom. We can choose recipes out of our cookbooks or make up something as we go along. Not long ago David made cinnamon pork chops. They turned out all right and everyone ate one. But next time David cooks, we'll ask him to make something else.

When Dad has had a rough week at work, we cook special dinners for him. Mom gets down the good china and glasses. We put a tablecloth and candles on the table. We even light the candles. Sometimes we make something really simple like pancakes. Other times we make our own recipes and Mom helps—but only if we need her.

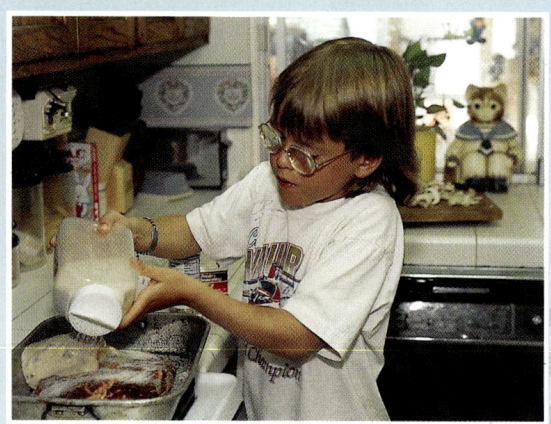

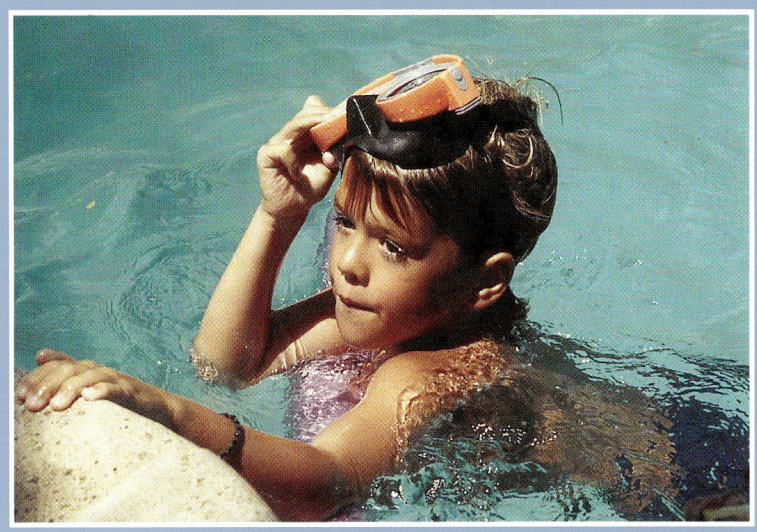

THREE YEARS AGO we moved into a bigger house. That's when we got our own bedrooms. Our bedrooms are our private spaces. We're careful about who we let into our rooms. If someone makes a mess in my room and doesn't pick it up, it's my responsibility to do it. We don't like cleaning up someone else's mess.

For our birthday we have one big party. We eat one big cake. We could have separate birthday parties and do different things if we wanted. But we like having a pool party together—swimming, barbecuing hamburgers, and playing with our friends.

A couple months before our birthday, we start making plans. We compromise on some parts of the party. Last year David wanted a dinosaur theme, but Donny had another idea. So David said, "Let's trade. If I can have dinosaur decorations, you can pick the flavor of cake." David and Donny agreed. A baker made our cake. He decorated it with a purple dinosaur for David, a blue dinosaur for Donny, and a red dinosaur for me. We had dinosaur plates, cups, and streamers.

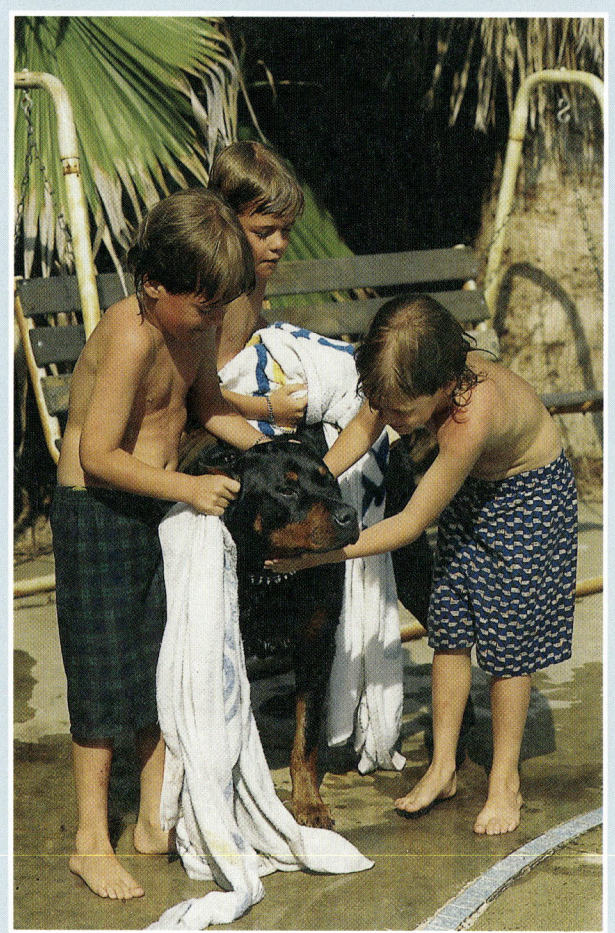

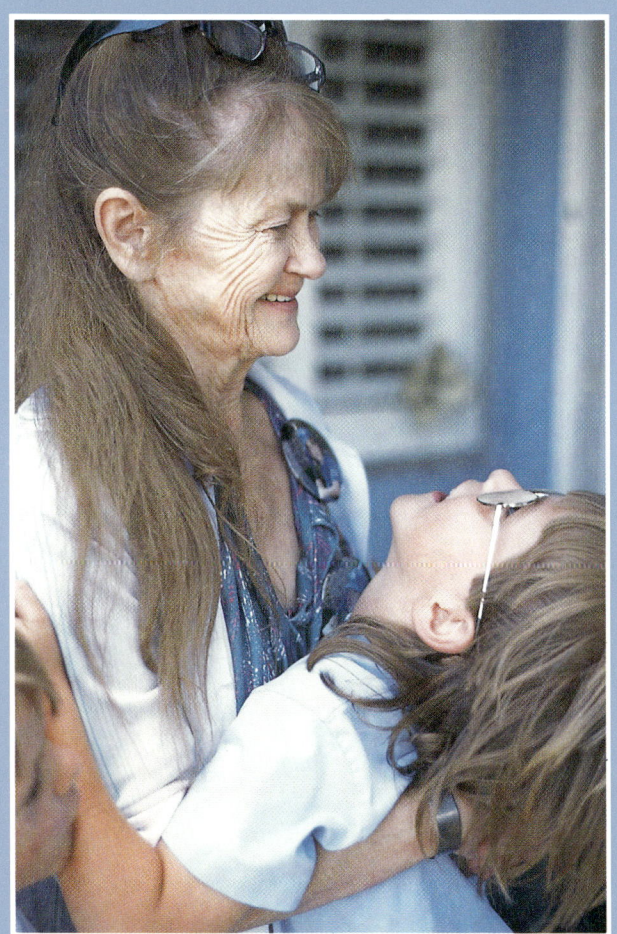

Each of us can invite only five friends from school. If Donny wants six of his friends at the party, he'll ask David and me how many friends we're planning to invite. Then we'll think about it. If one of us plans to ask just four friends, we may let Donny use one of our invites. We usually work it out by trading. But if David and I each want five friends, Donny will have to invite only five friends, too. We also invite our cousins and family friends. Grandma comes, too. It's one BIG party.

Before Mom and Dad buy us presents, they ask each of us what we'd like. They don't lump us together. They treat us as individuals. Mom and Dad say that just because we're identical triplets doesn't mean we have to like the same things. If Donny wants to go to the skating rink and David wants to do something else, that's okay. I don't really like motorcycles. So if Dad gives Donny and David a ride on his motorcycle, then Dad takes me for a special trip in his car.

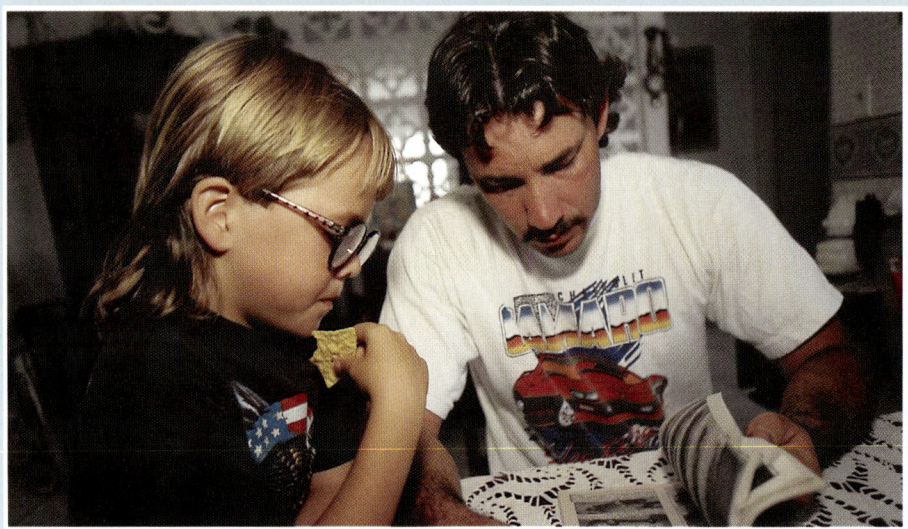

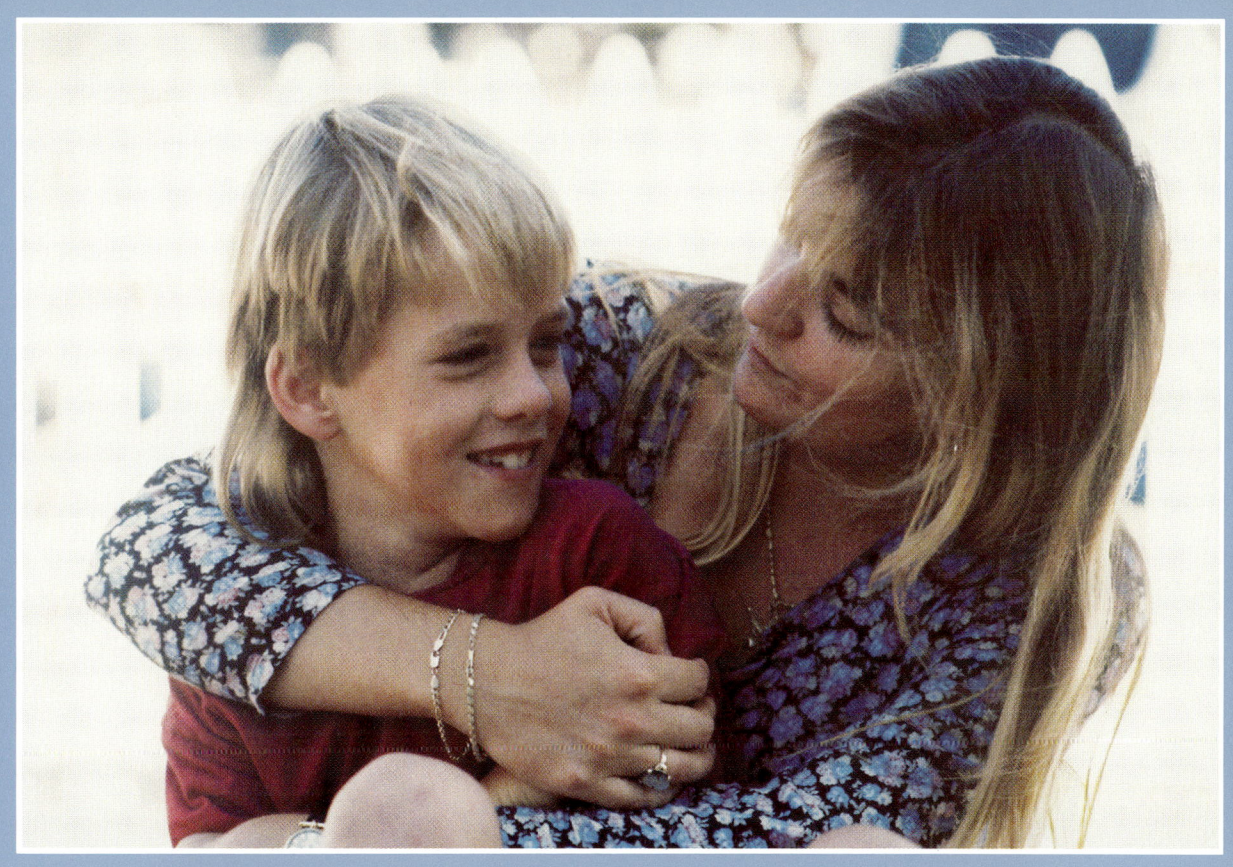

When David, Donny, or I want to be alone with Mom, she'll ask Dad to watch the other kids. We might take a walk, read a story, or do an art project together. Sometimes we go into the bedroom and just talk. Each of us spends time alone with Mom and Dad in different ways.

ON AN ORDINARY DAY, we wear our favorite colors—
purple, blue, and red. In school we put artwork on the walls
and study butterflies in our classes. At home we feed Edgar
and Inga and get wet kisses in return. And in Scouts we
work on derby cars and salute the flag with pride.

In the bathroom mirror, we see three different faces and
wonder why so many people can't tell us apart. When the
doorbell rings, we answer the door. If our friend calls us by
our names, we smile and say, "You're right."

"I'm David."

"I'm Donny."

"I'm Darren."

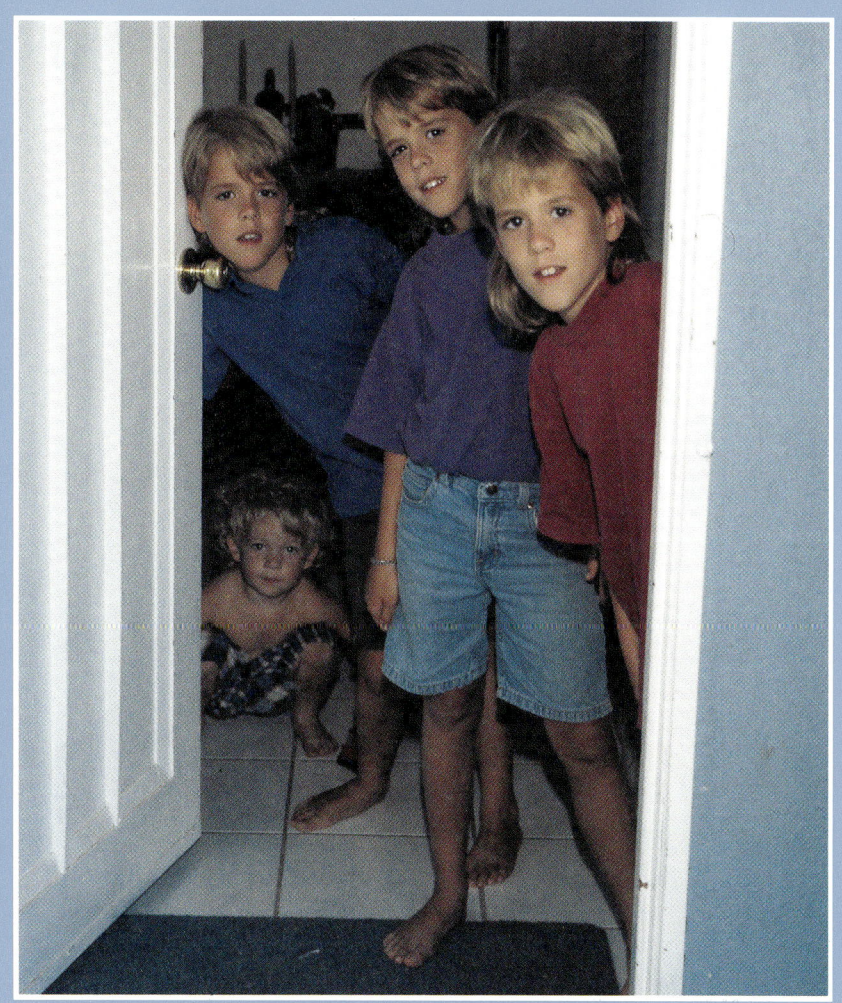

DAVID

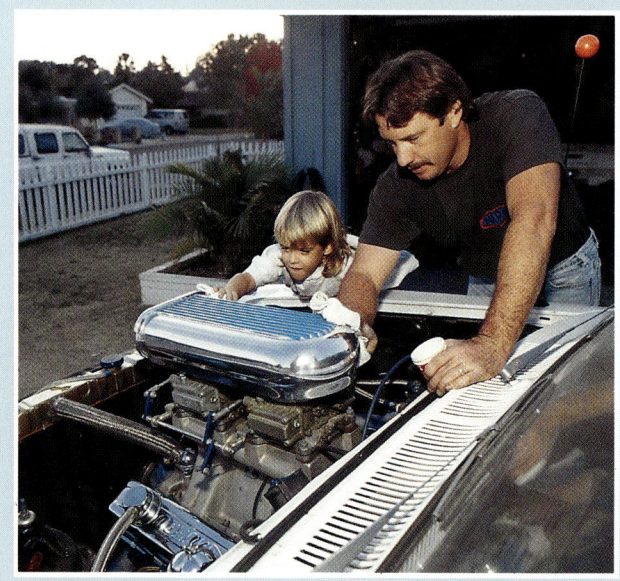

I like being a triplet because I have two friends to play with.

I like drag racing best because it is loud and we get to play in the pits. All of the family gets to come. We get to picnic lunch. My dad's car is cool because it goes fast and he always wins. I love my dad.

I like gluing, cutting, and drawing. I like to draw parrots because they're colorful, and clowns because they're funny.

I like it on Saturdays because I have a day off from school. Then I get to sleep in late and I get to watch a movie. I like movies that are scary and have lots of action.

Today is my mom's birthday. My wish is for my mom to have a good birthday party. My magic wish for the world is for everyone to have peace. No more wars.

DONNY

I'm a triplet. A triplet is a boy who has two brothers that look just like him. I kind of like being a triplet. I'm taller. I don't feel very well when grown-ups just call out our names. They go, "Donny, David, Darren."

I like camping because we get to play in the river and we get to sleep in our tent. We get to build a fire and roast marshmallows. We get to play in the sun.

I like writing, reading, and making a book.

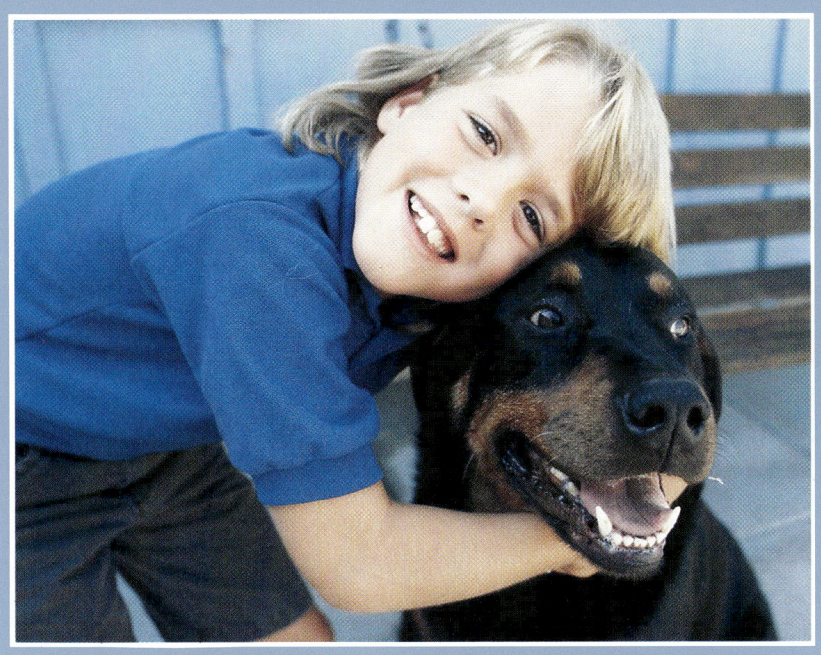

My favorite day was when we went to Disneyland. We stayed there for two days. The best part was going on the Roger Rabbit ride and Pirates of the Caribbean.

I wish I had a genie to clean my room. My wish for the world is that people would stop cutting down trees.

DARREN

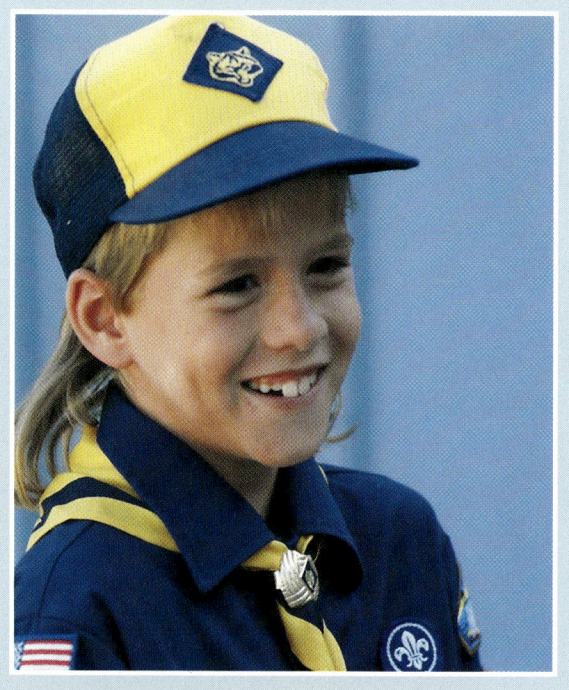

I like being a triplet because we get to trick
the teachers.

I like Cub Scouts. I get to play with my friends.
We are going on a camping trip and are having
a fish fry. I get to wear a cool uniform with

patches, a hat, and a neckerchief. Our friends, Eric and Kevin, are in our pack.

I like math and making projects like ants. To make an ant you get a piece of paper and you draw your best ant and color it in. Then you paste it on another piece of paper.

I liked Halloween last year. We got a lot of candy. We were all mouses, but I can't remember their names.

I wish I could turn into anything I want. For the world I wish there were no bad people and everyone would recycle.

Information about
MULTIPLE BIRTHS

A woman becomes pregnant when an egg that grows in her body joins with a sperm from a man. When the egg and sperm unite, the egg is fertilized. The fertilized egg develops into an embryo, which later becomes a baby.

Mothers usually give birth to only one baby at a time. But if a mother gives birth to two or more babies at the same time, it is called a "multiple birth." Multiple births include twins (two babies), triplets (three babies), quadruplets (four babies), quintuplets (five babies), and sextuplets (six babies).

Twins are the most common type of multiple birth in the world, occurring about once in every 89 births. Triplets occur about once in every 7,900 births and quadruplets about once in every 705,000 births.

There are two types of multiple births, *fraternal* and *identical.* Fraternal multiple births develop from two or more separately fertilized eggs. Each baby has a unique set of genes. Genes are the parts of a cell that shape characteristics such as eye color, hair color, and height. Fraternal babies may be all boys, all girls, or boys and girls. Fraternal babies usually don't look any more alike than other brothers or sisters in the same family.

Identical multiple births occur when a single fertilized egg splits in half, forming two embryos. After this first division, each embryo can divide again and again. Two, four, six, or eight embryos can start from one fertilized egg. Each embryo has the potential to grow, but probably only some will develop into a baby. It is hard for multiple embryos to develop because of problems such as lack of nutrients and not enough space to grow.

Since identical babies have the same genetic makeup, they are always *all boys* or *all girls*. Their hair and eye color are the same. Facial features, height, and weight are nearly the same. Identical babies even have the same blood type. Their footprints are similar, too. But their fingerprints are always unique. Identical babies are so much alike, it's hard to tell them apart.

Fraternal births vary according to ethnic origin. These births occur most often among people of African descent and least often among people of Asian descent.

The occurrence of identical multiple births is about the same throughout the world. The average chance of being an *identical twin* is 1 in 260. And the average likelihood of being an *identical triplet,* like David, Donny, and Darren, is 1 in 70,000.

Scientists have learned that genes play an important role in determining traits like height, weight, blood pressure, speech patterns, and gestures. That's why David, Donny, and Darren are very much alike and will continue to be throughout their entire lives.

Glossary

egg—a woman's reproductive cell, which can develop into a baby if it is united with a sperm

embryo—(EM-bree-oh) a developing baby in the first eight weeks of life

fertilization—(fur-tuh-luh-ZAY-shun) the joining of an egg from a woman and a sperm from a man

fraternal—(fruh-TER-nuhl) a term used to describe babies that have developed from two or more separately fertilized eggs. Fraternal babies do not look exactly alike because they have different genes.

genes—small parts of a cell that determine human characteristics like height and hair color

identical—(eye-DEN-tih-kuhl) a term used to describe babies that have developed from one fertilized egg that splits in half. Identical babies look alike because they have identical genes.

multiple birth—two or more babies born at the same time

quadruplets—(kwah-DROO-plits) four babies born at one birth

quintuplets (kwin-TUH-plits)—five babies born at one birth

sextuplets—(seks-TUH-plits) six babies born at one birth

sperm—a man's reproductive cell, which can develop into a baby if it is united with an egg

triplets—three babies born at one birth

twins—two babies born at one birth

Resources for PARENTS

National Organization of Mothers of Twins Clubs, Inc. (NOMOTC)
P.O. Box 23188
Albuquerque, NM 87192-1188
(800) 243-2276 or (505) 275-0955
On-line address: http://www.parentsplace.com/readroom/momsoftwins

Triplet Connection
P.O. Box 99571
Stockton, CA 95209
(209) 474-0885
On-line address: http://www.inreach.com/triplets

Twins Magazine
5350 S. Roslyn Street, Suite 400
Englewood, CO 80111
(800) 821-5533
On-line address: http://www.twinsmagazine.com

Twin Services, Inc.
P.O. Box 10066
Berkeley, CA 94709
(510) 524-0863
On-line address: http://www.parentsplace.com/readroom/twins

Photo Key *(left to right, or top to bottom)*

Front cover David, Donny, Darren

1 David, Darren, Donny

4 Donny, Darren, David

6 David, Darren, Donny

7 David, Donny, friend, Darren

8 David, Donny, Darren

9 Darren, friend

11 Darren, David, Donny

12 Pauly, Donny

13 *Back row:* Mom, Dad
Center row: Donny, Darren, David
Front: Pauly

14 Donny, Mom, David, Darren
(with Edgar and Inga)

15 Friend, David

16 Teacher, friend, Donny, friend

17 Donny

18 *Left photo:* Darren
Right photo: Darren, Pauly

19 David, Pauly

21 David, Darren, Donny

22 David

23 David

24 David, Darren, Donny
(with Edgar)

25 Grandma, Darren

26 Donny, Dad

27 Darren, Mom

29 *(From bottom left)*
Pauly, Donny, David, Darren

30 David, Dad

33 Donny (with Edgar)

34 Darren

Back cover *(From bottom left)*
Donny, Darren, Mom, David,